REFLECTIONS ON THE C-WORD

Reflections

For Bryan and Gerda,

on the **C-WORD**

At the centre of the cancer labyrinth

CAROL MATTHEWS

HEDGEROW PRESS

2007

With all good wishes,

Carol

Library and Archives Canada Cataloguing in Publication

Matthews, Carol, 1942-
    Reflections on the c-word: at the centre of the cancer labyrinth/ Carol Matthews (author); Jennifer Waelti-Walters (illustrator)

ISBN 978-0-9736882-5-2 (pbk.)

1.Matthews, Carol, 1942– Health. 2. Breast–Cancer–Patients–Religious life. 3. Breast–Cancer–Patients–Canada–Biography. I. Waelti-Walters, Jennifer, 1942– II. Title

RC280.B8M38 2007   362.196'994490092   C2007-903951-0

Published by
Hedgerow Press,
P.O. Box 2471,
Sidney, B.C. V8L 3Y3
hedgep@telus.net
www.hedgerowpress.com

Cover and text design: Frances Hunter
Photography: Robbyn Gordon
Author photograph by Mike Matthews

Printed and bound in Canada by Friesens
on 100% post consumer recycled paper

To
Dr. John Carr,
Dr. Elizabeth Feick
and Dr. Elaine Wai
for their excellent care,
to Connie, Jo and Sharon
for inspiration, and to the
family and friends who
see me through.

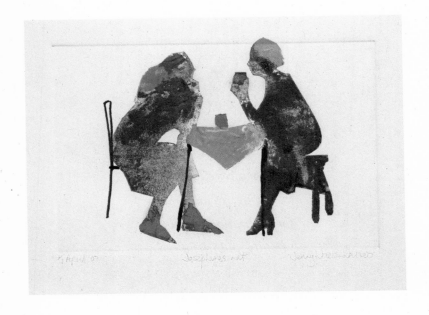

Talking

Contents

The Labyrinth

The first labyrinth I encountered was at Grace Cathedral in San Francisco many years ago. My husband and I were staying at a charming little boutique hotel not far from the Cathedral and enjoying the elegance of the city and of the hotel with its art deco furnishings, the good California wine served by the fireside each evening, and the big bowls of local apples at the front desk. It was by chance that I wandered into the Cathedral one morning to look at the famous stained glass windows. On this bright autumn day, the sun cast moving shafts of colour through the windows onto the church walls and on the barefoot people who circled around on the tapestry labyrinth at the centre of the hall. The scene was very California, I thought, very San Francisco, and quite beautiful. My husband waited outside while I took off my shoes and tentatively entered the labyrinth but I made only a few turns before going out to join him, having decided that the labyrinth was not for me.

A decade later, on a trip to France, I saw the Chartres Cathedral with its magnificent rose windows beaming their kaleidoscope of colour over the black and white stones of the labyrinth that was laid in the church floor in about 1220. I'd read that this eleven-circuit labyrinth, sometimes called the "Chemin de Jerusalem," served as a substitute for an actual pilgrimage to Jerusalem. On the day of our visit, though, the floor was covered with chairs and I later learned that it's only on certain days that the chairs are removed to allow people to walk the labyrinth. I sat in the great, dark hall and the organ sounded, huge chords resonating throughout the cathedral, great deep bass notes seeming to rise up from those old stones. When the immense doors were flung open so that sunlight streamed through, I tried to picture what it would have been like for a medieval pilgrim, perhaps after a tiring journey along the River Eure, to enter this enormous Gothic cathedral and walk the concentric circular flagstone path under those luminous windows. I could not imagine it.

A few years later, while I was a dean at Malaspina University-College, I attended a workshop at St. Paul's Anglican church in the West End of Vancouver. Called "The Labyrinth and the Art of Leadership" and led by two educators and an Anglican priest, this session proposed that the reflective practice of labyrinth walking was a valuable leadership tool. In walking the labyrinth, they said, busy administrators were able to let go of some of the superficial things that occupied so much of our attention and get in touch with the deeper purpose of our work. In the years that followed, I walked that labyrinth several times and found it to be helpful.

It was not until I learned that I had cancer, though, that I discovered the real value of the labyrinth as a tool for meditation, reflection, and self-discovery. It has kept me grounded throughout some difficult times. As Rev. Lauren Artress, Honorary Canon of Grace Cathedral, has said, walking the labyrinth teaches us how to quiet the mind. She describes the labyrinth as a "meandering but purposeful path" and says that the lesson is to trust the path.

Although there is no prescribed way in which one should walk the labyrinth, Artress speaks of the three R's: releasing, receiving, and returning. As you enter the labyrinth, you may begin to let go of details of the day-to-day world. Standing in the rosette, or the centre of the labyrinth, you may be open to illumination. On the path out, as you leave the labyrinth and return to the larger world, you may take with you the understanding that you've received. What I have taken from the labyrinth is nothing more than a framework that lets me reflect on questions that matter to me. That, and a fleeting sense that illumination is possible. It's enough.

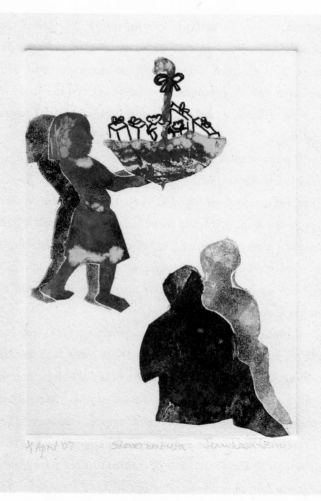

The Shower Umbrella

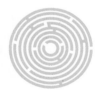

Remembering

AUNTIE MABEL WASN'T A BLOOD RELATIVE, only the cousin of my father's stepbrother's wife, but she was in many ways the heart of that side of the family. No marriage could take place and no baby be born without a shower at Auntie Mabel's house. As a young child I helped my mother decorate the umbrella that held the gifts at these showers. We would wind layer after layer of crepe paper, usually pink and mauve, or sometimes pale yellow, around an old umbrella frame and then, with our thumbs and forefingers, press each strip into little scalloped edges. "Like rose petals," my mother said.

Sometimes I helped make tea sandwiches, the proper kind: rolled sandwiches with olives in the centre, ribbon fingers filled with cream cheese and chopped maraschino cherries, and checkerboard sandwiches with alternating brown and white squares of bread. We wrapped them tightly in waxed paper and stored them in our refrigerator until they were transported to Auntie Mabel's, where they were arranged in thin slices on Auntie Mabel's beautiful old Wedgewood and Spode china plates.

It was my job to arrange cookies and cake on Auntie Mabel's two-tiered, flowered Royal Winton serving plate. I was, she said, the only person who could arrange cookies so beautifully; she herself was never able to do it quite so attractively. There were almost always Peak Frean biscuits and I would carefully alternate the long, thin, chocolate bourbon cookies with the oblong lemon puffs and the round, jam-centred ones which were my favourite. Often there were little tarts filled with Auntie Mabel's own "lemon cheese," an irresistible thick yellow custard which she made every year and stored in small glass jars until it was needed to fill tarts or, occasionally, to be spread on toast.

After the presents were opened, there would be a bit of a sing-song, usually when the men arrived to drive the women home, and Auntie Mabel would ask me to play a few songs on the piano, folk songs like "Early One Morning" and "Londonderry Air." If the men were singing, there would be "In Cellar Cool" and maybe "Old Man River." Auntie Mabel played the piano quite well and I was just learning, but she would excuse herself periodically, saying that her arthritis was acting up. And at some point I would be allowed to wind up and turn on the musical cigarette box which played "Do Ye Ken John Peel" while red-coated hunters and their hounds stood at attention as the box slowly opened to reveal a dozen cigarettes.

At the end of the evening Auntie Mabel always packed up cakes or cookies for us to take home. Once she gave us a whole tray of cream puffs but on the way home my mother insisted on throwing them into the garbage because she'd seen that they'd been sitting out on the counter all day and she was sure the cream would have turned. Couldn't we even just try them to see if they were all right? I asked. I wouldn't mind if they'd turned a little, I said. My mother said no, these things could be deadly, and we could all end up with food poisoning. It was ridiculous, she said, that Auntie Mabel kept on using that old icebox instead of getting a proper refrigerator.

I remember staying overnight there with my brother, and playing three-handed cribbage on Auntie Mabel's elk-antler cribbage board. Her dog Lucky, a fat black cocker spaniel, sat at our feet when we had tea, and Auntie Mabel fed him cookies and saucers of milk. In the morning she sent my brother and me out to the tiny garden to pick raspberries, dispatching Lucky to waddle along beside us. When we brought the raspberries in, she divided them into two sky-blue bowls, covered them with cream, and served them to us along with slabs of toast that were spread thickly with her sweet, tangy, golden yellow lemon cheese.

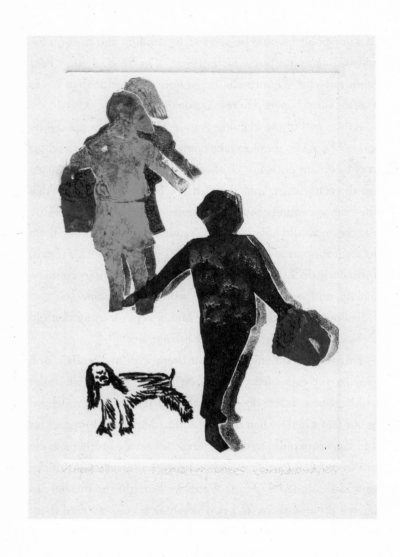

Picking Raspberries

When I was about nine years old, Auntie Mabel moved up to the Sunshine Coast to share a cottage with her recently widowed cousin. I didn't see her as often after that, but I went there for summer visits a couple of times with my mother. We slept in the guest room with its multi-coloured afghans and the bookcase filled with John Galsworthy and Lloyd C. Douglas novels. Down the hall Auntie Mabel and her cousin, Auntie Susie, shared a twin-bedded room, each with a bedside table covered with a lace doily, Auntie Susie's featuring her ornately framed wedding photograph, and Auntie Mabel's the photograph of an earnest-looking young man in a World War One uniform.

My mother told me that Auntie Mabel had never married because the man she had loved had been killed in the war. I tried to imagine Auntie Mabel being married, but I could not. She was pleasant-looking—bright blue eyes, and a cheerful, crooked smile—but her face looked a bit doggy to me, maybe because of the jutting chin and the little pug nose. Or perhaps it was just that she'd grown to look like Lucky, the way people and dogs do after living together for many years.

Sometime during the summer before my twelfth birthday Auntie Mabel began to stay with us for a few days every month. About that time my parents decided to move me to an upstairs bedroom. The large room that had been mine became a guest room, which was where Auntie Mabel stayed whenever she was in town. By then Lucky had died, and Auntie Mabel looked older and sadder, but she never failed to bring along a jar of lemon cheese and, if it was summer, a box of her fresh raspberries which were always somewhat mashed up in the transporting.

I can't now quite remember when this thing happened, but I know it must have been June or July, because my mother had made summer pudding on the second evening of Auntie Mabel's visit. It was the best thing you could do with mashed raspberries, she said. I thought it marvelous to see the way, after being refrigerated overnight with a brick to press it into the mold, the pudding was turned out as a perfect dome in which the raspberry juice had soaked right through the white bread, turning it a vibrant, marbled, purplish red.

Perhaps it was a nightmare that woke me, or perhaps it was the second helping of summer pudding, but I came downstairs to go to the bathroom in the middle of the night and surprised Auntie Mabel as she stood in front of the washbasin. Naked to the waist, she was rubbing a yellow ointment into the deep red lesions and craters on what was barely recognizable as a breast. I felt my stomach lurch and turned away as I heard my Auntie Mabel say, "Oh, my dear, I'm so sorry, I should have locked the door."

Nothing could bring me to look at Auntie Mabel at breakfast the next morning. I turned down the toast with its glistening, sickening lemon cheese, and I escaped to school without hugging anyone goodbye. The thought of my emerging breasts

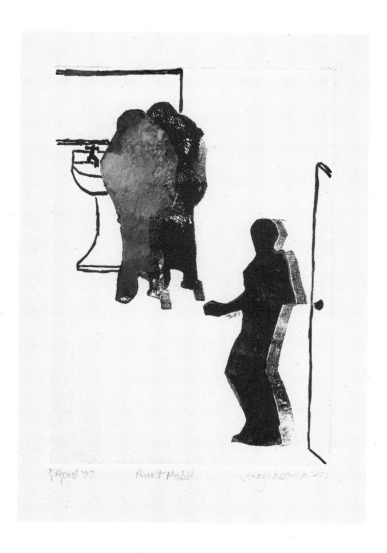

Auntie Mabel

pressing close to my aunt's body after what I had seen in the mirror was insufferable. After school that day my mother tried to talk to me about what had happened. She said Auntie Mabel was worried that I'd been upset and she wanted to apologize for leaving the door open. I brushed it off, pretending I didn't know what my mother was talking about.

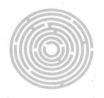

Discovering

SEVERAL WEEKS AGO I'd heard from a friend who had a scare with a lump in her breast that had only been detected through a mammogram. That's what prompts me to make the appointment. Out of the blue I find myself thinking of Auntie Mabel, who died from breast cancer five decades ago. No mammograms back then. I wonder whether she'd even had any friends who would talk about such intimate matters. I suppose she might have talked a bit with my mother, since they were both nurses, but as far as I know not much of a personal nature was spoken. I don't believe I ever heard anyone mention the words "breast cancer" in those days.

It's just a week before Christmas when the telephone call comes. With my daughter and her family arriving in a few days I don't want to cast a pall over the holidays so I set the follow-up appointment for just after Christmas. The person who arranges the appointment tells me that they get about six callbacks a day, and very often these situations don't require any further follow-up. A letter from the cancer clinic comes along with the Christmas cards and it too is intended to be reassuring. Of all the repeat X-rays, it says, a full 94 percent produce results that indicate that no treatment is required. So only 6 percent of the callbacks are in trouble? But wouldn't I buy a raffle ticket with a 6 percent chance of winning? And wouldn't my age, my weight, my general lack of fitness increase those odds?

My granddaughter Charlotte is sick with flu and has a very high fever on Christmas Eve, but she bounces back Christmas morning. My husband and I get up early to turn on the tree lights and put the Christmas music on and then we go back to bed to read until the others wake up. We want it to be magical when Charlotte comes in and discovers the stockings, but she heads straight for our room, wide-eyed and somber.

"Merry Christmas, Charlotte," I say. "Did Santa come?"

"No," she shakes her head.

"Didn't he fill the stockings?"

"No, he didn't. I looked all around. I even looked behind me but he was not there."

Somehow she'd had the idea that she'd be able to see him in person. When I take her to see the filled stockings under the tree she lights right up and sits down with our dog, Victor, to help him find the treats in his small stocking.

It is a joyful day. This house is a happy place for Charlotte. It has, I reflect, most of the features that Auntie Mabel's little house had: a doting elderly lady, a dog, a piano, some singsongs and lots of cookies. The old woman here has a husband, the dog is more vigorous and we lack that amazing music box, but many features are the same.

Charlotte will not always choose to be with us. Children grow up and their interests change. These days, I reflect, are the halcyon days. In fact, this is the actual halcyon period, the one week before and one after the solstice. These are the kingfisher days, the time of year when the seas were thought to be calm and the kingfishers could build floating nests made of fish bones on the sea and the female and her eggs would drift on the tranquil sea amidst becalmed winds. Halcyon is the classical name for the kingfisher and the halcyon days are supposed to be a time of joy, peace and prosperity. Will we all look back on this Christmas as a time when life was good? Before the world changed?

On December 28th, my husband drives me to the hospital and accompanies me to the area where they do the mammograms. Follow the yellow dots, the person at Information tells me, and indeed, just like at IKEA, there are yellow circles on the floor to lead me through the maze.

The technician asks me to take off the top part of my outfit, never mind about my earrings and glasses, put a hospital gown over my skirt, and then go to her office which has a pink ribbon on the door. The pink ribbon seems ominous. I know it is well-intended, but I dislike that frilly frivolous demarcation of breast cancer as a shared female experience that creates a pathological kind of bonding.

The technician is pleasant, professional yet open, and shows me on the X-rays the small dark spot on my right breast that had not been there in the previous pictures. She takes several more X-rays and then leaves me while she goes to talk to the radiologist.

The woman doing the ultrasound is less upbeat and has dark circles under her eyes. It must be tiring work, searching and searching for signs of cancer. She spends some time going over my breast again and again, peering at the screen, and then says she also is going to talk to the radiologist.

The radiologist introduces himself and we shake hands, although I don't quite catch his name. He too explains that there is something there that hasn't been in previous mammograms. He says whatever is there is a very small thing, only a speck, and even if it is cancerous it should be possible to deal with it easily. That's how we like it, he says, when it's very small like this. But he thinks it would also be a good idea to do a needle biopsy right now so that if it turns out to be something that is really a problem they can move things much more quickly. It's your choice he says, but I agree that we should do something immediately. What's the point of waiting?

It isn't a painful process, a quick freezing and then the moving around of the needle while he watches it on the screen. We talk about things while he does this. About the course I am scheduled to teach, about how I used to work in this hospital, decades ago, before working at the college. About how things change. The college, the hospital. It takes a couple of times before he is happy with the sample.

"Try not to worry," he says. "It really is very small." If I have swelling on my breast, a package of frozen peas will help, the technician tells me as I put my clothes back on. Swelling? Maybe, she says, because he sure did a lot of wiggling in there with that needle.

The next questions are who to tell and when. I consider talking to my daughter, but she will worry too much. It's bad timing, with her just starting to teach her first college-level credit course. And I've promised to be available for babysitting every week if she needs me. Will I be able to keep that promise?

I don't need to tell my daughter until after I have seen the doctor and know better what's ahead. Family? Friends? Colleagues? That's something to think about. Some obviously not, because they will talk too much or make too much fuss about everything. Anyway, I can't tell anyone else until I first tell my daughter. Meanwhile, I need to carry on and try to do healthy things.

The next morning I see that the bruise on my breast has formed a perfect "C." Every Christmas I make a little book of drawings and verses for Charlotte. The book I made this Christmas was about the alphabet, and the letter C gave me one of my drawings, a picture in which Charlotte and I are upside down and the verse says

> *C is for Charlotte, and Carol, and Christmas.*
> *If you didn't have us, you surely would miss us.*

If I were doing it now, I might think of different verses.

> *C, carcinoma, it sounds very pretty,*
> *but it isn't a word you should use in a ditty.*

Like belladonna, beautiful and deadly. If I were doing it today I might write

> *C is for Christmas and Carol and Cancer.*
> *For some kinds of questions, there isn't an answer.*

A Way Through

THE GRANITE FACE OF THE OLD CHURCH wears its age more gracefully than do the people inside the church hall. I labour up the stairs behind a wraithlike woman who has to stop at the door to take a deep breath before entering the labyrinth, which is on the upper floor. The hall is hushed, except for an early music CD playing in the background. Three people occupy the centre of the labyrinth: a barefoot, grey-haired man in a weathered beige tracksuit, a plump, middle-aged woman wearing a pink fleece sweatshirt and a dark navy woollen skirt, and a woman of indeterminate age in a purple yoga outfit, bent over in a crouching dog position, forehead touching the floor in front of her. I wonder, are we all ailing? All bringing lost hopes or hopeless cases?

I'm glad when my daughter turns up. She wears narrow black pants, high-heeled boots, a scarlet turtleneck and a long black coat with a red and orange scarf looped twice around her neck. Anyone would agree that she radiates good health, gives off strong vibrant energy.

She has come to offer me support, even though I told her that she needn't. Oh, I want to walk the labyrinth for myself anyway, she replied.

I'm walking the labyrinth today as a way to reflect on the surgery I am going to have next week. This ancient walking meditation, with its meandering path on which one makes thirty-four turns and faces the centre thirteen times, may help me think about where I am, what's ahead, and how I will find the courage I need to make my way through it all. That's my focus as I enter the labyrinth.

A young girl with blotchy skin and baggy jeans and dirty red and white socks is on the path ahead of me. I remind myself to focus on my feet, on taking even, measured steps while following the one-way path, and let the labyrinth work its meditative magic. I'm aware of my daughter's presence when, having taken off her boots and coat, she stands behind me, allowing some space to grow between us, before she too enters the labyrinth.

Courage, I think, *courage*, and immediately the word *fear* comes into my mind. I go with the word. The word seems to bring about a change in chemistry, a thickening of the blood, a sudden sweetness in the saliva and a touch of vertigo. I've been telling people that I'm not afraid, but is that true? If I think of all the possibilities, how could I not be afraid? Unconsciousness, vulnerability, pain. What if I'm allergic to the anaesthetic, or if it doesn't work properly? Complications, bleeding or clotting. And things could turn out to be much worse than expected. The cancer may have spread everywhere, worming its way through my body like this twisting path I am traveling.

To die and face not being? I let my thoughts encounter every scenario until I come to the conclusion that it is the fear itself that is most to be feared. What each possibility brings, at its worst, is more fear.

Someone once told me that fear is given out to cowards and heroes in equal measure. I think of the people who are walking behind and ahead of me. We are all here for a reason, all no doubt trying to find a way to deal with something that is challenging us. The grey-haired man and the woman in pink have left the "rosette," the sacred centre of the labyrinth, where I now join the young girl and the yoga woman and stand inside one of the six petals, gathering my thoughts, hoping for some new awareness. Now another woman enters the labyrinth. She wears wide pants quilted in colourful, silky squares, a cape of similar construction, a splendid turban and an array of sparkling beads. Barefooted, she begins her walk with a languorous pace and a confident smile that suggests she will take this ritual many levels deeper, or higher—or to a different place—than the rest of us.

Awareness, I tell myself, is also one of the things I need to focus on over the coming weeks. Courage, awareness and a way of living with uncertainty. *Grace* perhaps is the best word for that. I want to develop an easy elegance in the way I will deal with the fear that is handed out equally to cowards and heroes.

My daughter has arrived beside me, but I am concentrating on the painting of the dark-skinned Mary Magdalen that hangs on the south wall. In her hand she holds a perfect white egg, the symbol of generativity and of the future. Looking at her, I realize just how much I want time to see my granddaughter grow up. *Enjoyment.* I want more time to enjoy the world and the people I love in it.

I almost laugh out loud when I realize that I have formed an acronym from the four things I am seeking. Courage, awareness, grace and enjoyment give me the word CAGE, which is so fitting for where I am on this path, figuratively and literally. Where we all are: me, my radiant daughter, the purple yoga lady and the spotty-faced girl who is now weeping silently, and those others who are winding their way outwards. We are all in this cage together, all on the same path. And the path out will be the same one that brought us here.

Walking the labyrinth has given me a few tools. First, there's the cage to carry—courage, awareness, grace, and enjoyment.

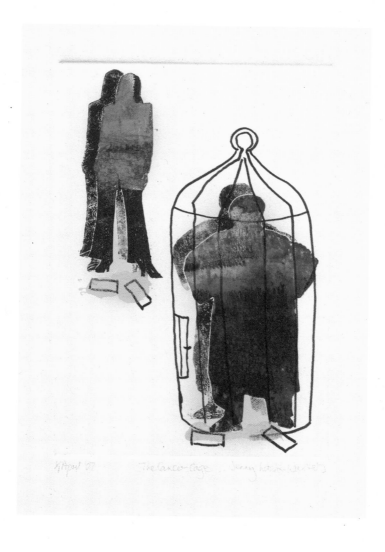

The Cancer Cage

And, then, in Saint Augustine's words, *"Solvitur ambulando."* Problems can be solved, or at least helped, by walking. And, as the Buddha said, "No one saves us but ourselves. No one can and no one may. We ourselves must walk the path."

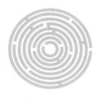

What Ails You?

PEOPLE RESPONDED VERY DIFFERENTLY when I told them that I was going to have surgery to have a malignant tumour removed. A lumpectomy—such an ugly word. My husband was the first person I told, and he didn't say a lot, but was predictably solid and somewhat more demonstrably concerned than I'd anticipated. I was apprehensive about telling my daughter because I thought it would be hard on her and that she'd probably be quite emotional. She was emotional, but she was also sensible, practical and supportive. My brothers and their children were like that too: calm, concerned, but positive.

An old friend, one who I thought might worry and fuss too much, said nothing. Well, in fact, she actually did say just one thing; she said, in an offhand way, that it seemed a lot of people feel very vulnerable when they find out they have cancer, even if the prognosis is quite good. "It makes them aware of their mortality," she said, "makes them feel their age and think about death even if it isn't a life-threatening situation." I said I thought I was already quite aware of my mortality and then we went on to talk about something else. She hasn't mentioned it again.

Some people insist that, although I sounded positive, I must be angry. Don't you think, "Why me? Why is this happening to me?" one friend asked. Well no, actually, I don't. Why not me? I'm surprised I've made it this far in my life without having had to face a few bad things. It's about time, that's what I think. You can only coast along as easily as I've done for so long.

A couple of my friends broke into tears and spoke at length about how upset they were. I tried to be reasonable and reassuring, talking about the early detection and the good prognosis, but I wanted to say, "Hey, this is *my* story. If anyone gets to cry, it should be me, shouldn't it?"

I guess there's no right way. Some people probably want their friends to be angry, or to cry, or to pretend nothing is happening. But what I liked best was having a number of friends simply say something like this: "Good God! I'm so sorry! When is your surgery? Is there anything I can do to help?" or, simply, "I'll be thinking of you." And I was pleased if they noted my positive energy and expressed confidence in a good outcome.

All the responses are fine. What matters is that people care, that they send their thoughts, energy and love. It's not the tradition in my family to speak about feelings of sadness, or fear, or vulnerability. Although we're all great talkers and it's often hard to get a word in edgewise at family gatherings and celebrations, when it comes to the real life and death issues we just don't say much. We love words in poetry and prose, but it's as though we don't think that words will help in these difficult, potentially emotional, situations and so we are silent.

But this time it's different for me. I've been thinking about the wounded Fisher King in the Grail legends, his spirit sick and sterile and his kingdom a wasteland. He hears and responds to Parsifal's question, *What ails you, friend?* It's the question that prompts an inner examination and a quest for wholeness, which is what the Grail story seems to mean. The search for that holy vessel is about spirit and completeness. The sick man answers the question, acknowledges that he is thirsty, drinks the water that he is offered, and is healed as a result. The world around him is restored to life and becomes productive and fruitful.

I don't want to make too much of this. I accept that illness can be a challenge to change and a journey to self-discovery. But I don't want to push the metaphor: I like to take it at the simplest level. Being asked the question, What ails you? and being willing to answer it and to accept nurture from others is helping me. I have taken the thoughts and wishes and love from others with me through this process and I find it helps.

I was moved when I heard that friends who are working in Cambodia right now, building shelter for the poorest of poor children, went to the highest temple in Angkor Wat on the day of my surgery. They said they would light candles in all four directions and send prayers from that ancient sacred place on the other side of the world. When the anaesthetist began her work, I thought about my good friends performing this ritual of love for me. It was a wonderful image to have in my mind as I lost consciousness.

Friends and neighbours have turned up with books and food and flowers. One friend has brought me flowers every week since I told her about the callback, and says she will keep on bringing more flowers each week until I am well again. A niece delivered a huge box of videos to divert me during my convalescence. My daughter brought a photograph of herself and my granddaughter to brighten my time at the hospital, as well as a light, citrusy cologne for my homecoming. One of her friends delivered a bundle of healthy homemade cookies and a tin of elegant, green tea bath cubes. Many, many friends told me they were sending their thoughts, love, white light, healing energy, and so on. A few said they were lighting candles for me. I haven't heard the results of the post-surgery biopsy but, in the meantime, all this support actually keeps my energy strong and my hopes high.

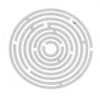

Spare Parts

My friend Jo, who lives on the other side of the country, has cancer too. She has been very ill but describes herself as "crawling back" and says that her "skin-flapping" body has decided to stick. She is eager to begin radiation treatment, but she has lost so much weight since her surgery that the doctors are reluctant to recommend treatment. On the telephone we joke about the irony of her having to drink milkshakes and eat chocolate bars and recall the days when we were always, as she would say in her soft Yorkshire accent, "slimming." We could not have imagined the time would come when additional calories were actually prescribed.

In fact, Jo was always slim and she was so lovely. I remember the day I met her, soon after she arrived in Montreal, one of those winter days when the world was dappled with snow and large white dots formed a lattice in front of our eyes, like the popcorn veils on the cocktail hats I used to wear when I was young. Jo's red hair was tucked up under her green hat and she was laughing. She had light green eyes and skin so white it was almost blue. She seemed to crackle with vitality.

"Wouldn't it be useful to have a few spare parts available for our Golden Age?" she says now, having heard about my breast cancer. "A leg here, a breast there, a few fine sheets of tissue to re-surface inner cavities?"

The truth is, we have ourselves become spare parts, I think. We've become unnecessary, *de trop*, out of the game. Nobody actually says this out loud, of course, but I've noticed that people speak to me differently when they know I have cancer. It's hard to pin it down but I can sense a slight difference in tone. They speak with concern, kindness and genuine feeling; I'm reminded of how I felt when I didn't make the grass hockey team or didn't make the finals for the music festival. Everybody would express their disappointment and concern but something had changed. I remember the hugs, the arms tossed around my shoulder, but I felt a rift growing between me and those others and thought that the rift wouldn't be there when they were just talking among themselves. They might say encouraging things to me—oh, you'll be able to play spare, you can still come to the games and the parties—but I knew I wasn't really one of them anymore. I was weakened. One of the wounded who had to sit the game out on the sidelines.

I thought I knew all about what it was like to be out of the game. Not just from those youthful experiences but from my more recent experience of taking early retirement. Once you take on the label "retired" people treat you a little differently. They start to call you "dear" a little more often and if you undertake any semi-serious activity they express astonishment and exclaim, "I thought you were supposed to be retired!" "Yes, but I'm afraid I still wake up in the morning," I had to exclaim to an old colleague I encountered recently.

The cancer business is different again and it ratchets everything up a couple of notches. You must endure not just being patronized but also being pitied. You've become something other, something diseased, cloaked in fear, and also, in a curious way, public property.

When I first became a college dean, I was surprised by the paradoxical effects that the mantle of position and power created. I hadn't known until then that it was possible for people to treat you with contempt and suck up to you at the same time. Cancer can create similar contradictions. I'm often puzzled to meet a response that seems to combine approach and avoidance. But I shouldn't be surprised. I've experienced it already.

Am I being hypersensitive? Maybe. I feel the cancer has brought about a heightening of my awareness. I'm more acutely awake to undertones in speech and subtexts in words now, in the same way in which I can really taste a dark roast in my morning coffee, and a whiff of leather or a tincture of raspberries in the one glass of wine I allow myself each night.

Forty years ago, as a twenty-year old, I regularly made tracks through the snowy streets between my room on St. Mark Street to Jo's basement suite on St. Mathieu. We would sit at the small, round oak table which she had hand-sanded and oiled to a gleaming finish. Watching the snow fall behind the lace curtains and the scarlet geraniums that blossomed on Jo's street-level window sill, we drank thick instant coffee laced with cheap French brandy and talked of lovers, landlords, and future travels. Time stretched endlessly before us.

Now, as grandmothers, connected across the country by telephone wires, we speak of the precious things we have in lives that seem so dramatically foreshortened. We imagine a Montreal meeting that might take place if we both make it through our treatments, but mostly we celebrate the daily events in the small worlds of each of our homes. Between us, it is all essential. We are both absolutely present and engaged in our own game. The timing is critical, everything matters, and every moment counts. There are no spare parts.

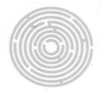

Grace Notes

I'VE NOW LEARNED THAT I'LL NEED to have another surgery to ensure a "wider margin" around where the tumour was. I'm taking it in good grace. I like and trust the surgeon, it will only be a day surgery and I heal quickly. It's a bit of a setback but I will handle it with courage, if not awareness, or grace.

I've been thinking about grace lately, not in the catechismal sense of a divine or sanctifying state but in terms of free and undeserved help, or as an unearned favour. This, of course, is what grace is. Simply a gift.

One day I was bragging to a friend about how much more disciplined and diligent I was than my husband and he said, "Yes, but Mike doesn't need discipline; he has grace." And it's true. He glides along, generally content, while I fret and worry and work. *Il se sent bien dans sa peau*, another friend said of him, and that's true too. He is easy in his skin, happy in himself.

Sometimes he dances around the house. I marvel at how graceful he can be, for such a large man, and I wonder why he has rarely wanted to dance in public. The other day he told me that he'd done an imitation of the waltz for his students, and I asked how one would do that, as opposed to dancing the waltz. "I can't dance," he explained. "I have no idea how to waltz, so I do an imitation." He chanted "Oom pah pah, oom pah pah," and twirled ferociously about the room. "I would call that a waltz," I told him, "not an imitation." But he insisted that he could not dance, that this was just something he did for his students. They split their sides laughing, he added.

Joy is a part of it too, a kind of exuberance. As Karl Barth, the Swiss theologian, said, "Laughter is the closest thing to the grace of God." The gift that we are given and also our appreciation for it. *Gracias. Grazie. Grace.*

I picture the way Victor, our dog, springs out of the house in the early morning, bounds from the deck, streaks along the path, his nose to the ground, as he unerringly follows the scent of a raccoon or a mink. He leaps through tall grasses like a dolphin, arc after arc, in one long fluid motion. Every movement is easy, elegant, and effortless.

My three-year-old granddaughter moves in much the same way. Her body is in constant motion but it is without thought

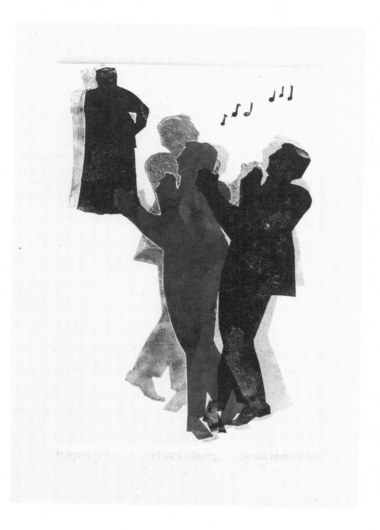

Mike's Waltz

or exertion. Running, squatting, rising or falling, every atom in her being seems to be perfectly balanced. Arms and limbs bend like rubber, flow like water. I'm not sure Samuel Taylor Coleridge was absolutely correct when he said, "How inimitably graceful children are in general before they learn to dance!" Charlotte already dances beautifully—but Coleridge was right to observe that there is beauty in the natural, unself-conscious movements of a child.

In her novel *Swamp Angel*, Ethel Wilson refers to an action which has "operative grace," one in which a person "seeing some uneasy sleeper cold and without a cover, goes away, finds and fetches a blanket, bends down, and covers the sleeper because the sleeper is a living being and is cold." The person does not need praise or thanks and the action is beautiful in combining posture and intention and self-forgetfulness.

Posture. Intention. Self-forgetfulness. My husband claims these are also present in the action of athletes. There is perfect efficiency and ease, he says, with nothing extraneous in it whatsoever, when a basketball player rises up, arcing a ball towards the hoop for a field goal. It is a beautiful and graceful action. I wonder if I can learn to discipline my spirit in this way.

Grace involves more than discipline. In its fullest form it has to do with an appreciation and acknowledgment for all that life has given us—life, creation, the natural beauty of the world. In his poem "The Peace of Wild Things," Wendell Berry writes that when he feels despair for the world he goes to lie down "where the wood drake rests in his beauty on the water, and the great heron feeds."

Like Berry, I find solace in watching the floating ducks and stalking herons feeding at the shore. When I despair about what the future holds for my child and my grandchild, I am comforted by the steady rise and fall of the ocean, the mysterious rhythms of the tides—ebb tides, neep tides, spring tides, even the falling tides. I remember what Annie Dillard said about looking at Tinker Creek: "It is the answer to Merton's prayer, 'Give us time!' It never stops…You wait for it, empty-handed, and you are filled."

The ocean too is unpredictably generous, bringing gifts of all kinds—shells, stones, every sort of sea creature dragged up from the deep. Often I see a seal surfacing close to shore, ducking down, playfully disappearing, and reappearing moments later. Once I saw three orcas, one and then another, and another, rise up in our little bay, taking my breath away with the power of their silent presence.

Grace is most simply a gift. Thus it also becomes that which is given, as my cancer is a given. It simply is and must be accepted. The fact that I must have another surgery is now a given and only that. It's just another thing and not a big thing, not on a large scale, when you look at the whole picture, although it is a gift I would have preferred not to receive.

The coming surgery is only an embellishment, like the grace notes my Auntie Mabel used to add to her piano performances, in true Victorian style. Grace notes and glissandos, the delicate turns and the long, flamboyant slides that added colour to an otherwise simple melody. That's what's ahead now, and it's not a major event. The long life that has been given to me is already in place and these next late episodes are not what it's all about.

There are two types of grace notes, I recall. Which is determined by how long they actually take to play. One type is called the *appoggiatura*, the leaning note, or so-called "time-taking ornament." The other is the *acciaccatura*, the crushing note, which has been called "the timeless moment." What lies ahead will be nothing more. It will be one thing or the other.

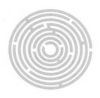

Back into the Labyrinth

I AM BACK AT THE LABYRINTH and this time I'm thinking about hope. It occurs to me that I'm a lot better at acceptance and endurance than I am at hope, yet I have a sense that it's important to stay hopeful, to have a vision of a successful recovery. It isn't that I am depressed—in fact I'm probably experiencing greater joy in small moments than ever before—but I just find it difficult to imagine a good outcome.

There are only a few people at the labyrinth and one of them is my dear niece with whom I will later go out for brunch. I'd hoped for live music but it is a silent walk today. I'm feeling cheerful. I mostly have a positive attitude, I've been told, although it sometimes seems to be a bit of a reproof. "Well, you really have a Good Attitude, don't you?" The implication is, perhaps, that I'm hiding something behind it, that maybe it's something I should "see somebody" about. Shouldn't I try to work through that Good Attitude and unleash the underlying rage and despair?

Most of my efforts have been focused on courage, something I haven't had much need of until now in my all too comfortable life. I can keep up a reasonable appearance of bravery, mostly by just thinking about it. Thinking about it is one of the things I do best and I have a pretty sensible approach. Courage and intelligence, those would be the linchpins, but if hope were also there, the acronym would be *chi* and that is exactly what I want: healing life energy that will help me survive this ordeal. CHI. This is better than the CAGE acronym.

Lately I hear a lot of people talking about "fighting" cancer. I read obituaries about people who have died after a "valiant battle" against cancer and I realize that wouldn't be me. I don't do battle very well. I'm better at finding my way around obstacles than I am at tackling them head-on. I don't like confrontations. I prefer simple avoidance or clever strategy. But I can't avoid this and I don't know what the strategy might be.

I've been reading Reynolds Price's memoir about his experience with spinal cancer. He talks about the tumour in his spine as an eel, and as a ravenous, alien twin he must fight and destroy. He envisions his own white blood cells surrounding and defeating the intruder. I've been unsuccessful in this kind of visualization, able only to imagine the renegade cancer cells as fast little insects like beetles or silverfish, darting into dark corners of the breast much too swiftly to be the object of any attack.

When you have cancer, everybody has a cancer story to tell you. Anyone with cancer will tell you this. Everyone has had a mammogram scare, or has sold daffodils for the cancer society, or done the Run for the Cure or has a mother-in-law who is still doing fine after cancer that was diagnosed as inoperable twenty-five years ago. Today I had a call from someone telling me about a woman whose doctor said that cancer was everywhere in her body and that she required immediate surgery, although the prognosis was not good. This woman went home, visualized like crazy, then insisted that more tests be conducted and, lo and behold, the cancer was gone! The woman actually felt the point at which the cancer disappeared, said my informant. She'd used the Pacman method of visualization, imagining the little creatures steadily munching away at her cancer cells. I googled "Pacman" and "visualization" and "cancer" and sure enough found something called "the Simonton method" of guided imagery which teaches cancer patients to picture armies of Pacman-like attackers gobbling up cancer cells.

So if my next biopsy report shows cancer, it'll be my fault.

My visualization skills suck, that's the problem.

No. Cancer sucks.

If I could relax and allow the *chi* energy to become a flow of spirit that is in harmony with the energy around it, maybe it could quietly contain and transform the rebel activities.

"Acceptance allows flowingness," someone told me. I am going to practise deep breathing and concentrating on acceptance. What will flow from this acceptance is not clear, however. Which side will the *chi* choose, me or the cancer?

The labyrinth is a good setting for envisioning flow. Within the circle, there is only flow, the winding path snaking its way to the centre and back. I catch a glimpse of my niece and admire her focus and her natural grace. I take pride in the good fortune of our family. Family and friends are finally what matter. *Family and friends, dear family, dear friends.* It is a mantra I repeat until I find myself thinking about begats. My mother and father begat three children, two sons and a daughter, all of whom married and begat, all in all, seven offspring. My husband's parents begat two sons, both of whom married and begat six children. From these thirteen came another generation of children, fourteen in all so far and likely more to come. Begats and more begats.

As in the labyrinth, I find that some are closer, some more distant, but the connection with all of them gives me great pleasure. And the intimacy with a few gives me deep delight. The thought that they and their children will carry on long after me makes my spirit rise. The sheer joy at the thought of it.

Here it is then. *Chi.* There is a moment, always, in the labyrinth where I feel the path flowing in both directions, inwards and outwards, forward and backwards. For an instant I seem to see those I love, my family and friends, as though from a great

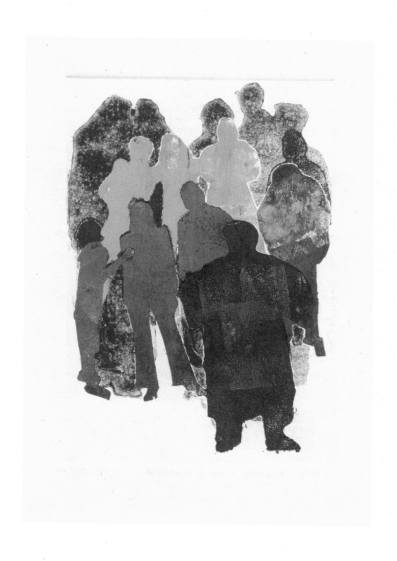

Importance of Family

distance, moving forwards and away from me, and I think, *It's OK, they will all carry on, I can let it go and leave them only my love and my strongest good wish for whatever lies ahead.* And at the same time I drift backwards, recalling my own childhood, remembering those I loved who are now gone.

Not long after that night when I saw Auntie Mabel in the bathroom, her situation worsened and within a few months she died. I think she must have requested there be no funeral. When I remember our last encounter, I feel sad for us both. We didn't know what to say to each other, had no way to speak about what had happened. In my book for Charlotte, I should have written

> *C is for Cheese, lemon cheese on your toast.*
> *If I had it now, that's what I'd like most.*

For now I will leave the labyrinth and go out for brunch with my own niece and I will revel in this relationship, this fortunate if unearned friendship. Later my husband and I will go for dinner with my daughter and her husband and their daughter. For now, that's as far as I can go. And as far as I need to go.

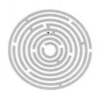

Radiating

"APRIL IS THE CRUELLEST MONTH," I announce to my husband as we drive towards the Victoria Cancer Clinic. "Not in Victoria," he replies, "it's the coolest." Grey skies turning blue, city streets transformed by blossoms and bulbs bursting into flower. Drifts of petals falling like pink snowflakes. Spirits rising. Spring, spring, spring, spring, spring. My first poem, at about eight years old, was:

> *Spring is here,*
> *Spring is here,*
> *Spring is the loveliest time of the year.*
> *Flowers are blooming,*
> *Children are gay.*
> *Everything's here for a wonderful day.*

I was very proud of this verse, especially when the Vancouver *Province*'s Tillicum Club chose to publish it, but my brother told me he did not believe I'd written it since, he claimed, a kid would never use the word "gay" in a poem, that was just something no kid would do.

Despite the spring season, my own spirits are less than gay as I brace myself for a week of intensive radiation therapy, two half-hour sessions per day for five days. I've been thinking about the word "radiate" and its many definitions. It can refer to sending out rays or waves, and it's also used to describe something that extends in straight lines from or towards the centre, as in spokes radiating from a wheel hub. The definition which seems most apt to me is the ecological one, which has to do with spreading into new habitats, diverging or diversifying.

I've been apprehensive about what it will be like to be surrounded by cancer patients, but as soon as I enter the building my anxiety diminishes. There's a gentle, accommodating slope to the ramp at the entrance of the Cancer Clinic, and the combination of wood, stone and natural landscaping is reassuring. Inside, the high ceilings, wide corridors and ample windows help to provide an airy atmosphere. Some people do look thin, frail, and a number of women are wearing those knitted caps that are designed for bald heads, yet it's a surprisingly cheerful place. I practise smiling, but I'm not by nature a smiler, being somewhat inclined to W.C. Field's approach: *Start each day with a smile, and get it over with.*

I try to imagine how I will adapt to this new habitat. Because the tumour was small, chemotherapy has not yet been proposed, so I will avoid some of the most unsettling aspects of treatment — the loss of hair, eyebrows, eyelashes, and the awful nausea. I'm grateful that I've been accepted into a research program in which my treatment will consist of accelerated partial breast irradiation. This means I'll have two sessions a day for one week, rather than the more usual format of one session a day for six weeks. I'm not sure that I'd have been able to endure that. It would have been hard to be away from home for so long, and I don't think I would have adapted well to the new habitat over the long-term. As it is, I will receive 38.5 units of radiation delivered to "the tumour bed" in ten treatments, morning and afternoon, over a period of only five days. My husband will drive me to Victoria, take me back and forth for each session, and stay with me through the week at the home of my brother and sister-in-law. I'm trying to see it as a kind of holiday.

I've been fitted for a sort of mold that will help me to stay still for the 30 minute treatments, and my breast has been tattooed with small dots to show the technicians where to focus the camera. I have a handle to grip onto so that I can stay in the right position, but it's difficult for me to stay immobile for so long. Somehow I'd had the idea that I was going to be placed in a tube of some sort, like the equipment used in some kinds of medical imaging processes, and I'm relieved to find that this is not the case. Even so, and pleasant and approachable though the radiation technicians are, I can't help feeling disempowered as I lie, prone and half-naked, on a stretcher while enormous, whirring machines circle around, flashing lights and emitting toxic rays.

There's a hint of the torture chamber about all this, and I find myself thinking about Viktor Frankl's memoir *Man's Search for Meaning*, about the kind of powerlessness he experienced in Auschwitz, where he was stripped of everything and everyone he loved. Frankl found that, even in these unspeakable circumstances, what he still possessed was the ability to choose his own thoughts. He believed our main purpose in life is to find meaning and said that, no matter how dire the circumstances, there are areas in which you can exercise control and choice.

Of course, my own situation is utterly different. I am here voluntarily and hoping to be helped, yet it is hard to escape the sense that one has become an object, powerless and no longer able to exert agency. I'm determined to exercise what choice I can, so I choose to use this half hour as a kind of concentrated thinking and planning time. I let myself wonder about the future, about where and how we should live, and I ponder over questions about whether or not we should move from our home on Protection Island and find a place that is lower maintenance and perhaps closer to medical services in the event that my condition worsens. I construct mental lists of the various pros and cons, trying to imagine how I might make the best use of my life in these later months and years.

Five days in the habitat of the Cancer Clinic will be more than enough for me. I wouldn't adapt well to a longer stay and so, again, I acknowledge my good fortune in having the option for short-term treatment. I'm a reclusive person with a limited capacity for diversification.

On the other hand, I have a great capacity for diversion and versification, and I am well-served by my friend Gerry who emails me a little ditty to encourage me on the first day of my treatment:

> *If the prospects of the day seem rather dismal*
> *And the week ahead is making you feel blue*
> *If your view of life is nothing but abysmal*
> *Then here's my little ditty just for you.*
> *Whether lying on your back or on your belly*
> *Take this thought— it's really quite profound*
> *To know with gratitude*
> *That you're inside the tube*
> *It could have been the other way around.*

45

I should let him know that the tube-like machine did not in fact materialize and things are going much better than I'd anticipated. I'd been warned that fatigue is to be expected but through the week of treatment I'm not unusually tired. I nap in the afternoon, between the two daily treatments, and then in the evening I'm ready to go out. My brother and sister-in-law have a large home, and they maintain an easy hospitality that makes it comfortable to be either reclusive or sociable. Towards the end of the week they get tickets for the four of us to see *Rigoletto*, which is beautifully staged and sung by Victoria's Opera Company, and full of viciousness and venom. The swarming of the courtiers abducting Rigoletto's daughter is chilling, as is Gilda's demise, being slaughtered in the sack and then reappearing as a spirit to sing her last words. Later that night I am unable to sleep, thinking about evil, about what a longstanding human tradition it has been.

Maybe my little granddaughter is right. "There are too many humans here!" she started to announce when she was barely three years old. "Will the humans please leave now?" she would ask. Charlotte likes, in something like this order, puppies, kittens, dogs, cats, horses, sheep, lambs, dolphins, whales, birds, toads, turtles, rabbits, moles and mice. She's "not crazy about" the idea of stoats, weasels and rats, but she'd probably like them too, if she met them face to face.

Charlotte knows the name of every dog she has ever met, but refers to their owners as, simply, "Skeena's person" or "Odie's person." She spends a lot of time on all fours, using her hands like paws and imitating animal behaviour. It isn't that she anthropomorphizes animals; rather, she zoomorphizes herself. The bottom line is that she likes animals more than people. Much more.

Lately, sometimes, I find myself sharing her perspective. There was a time when humans were in the minority, and some things may have been better back then. There wasn't a lot of pollution in those early days, or global warming, or avian flu, or AIDS, and there was no immediate threat from depletion of the earth's resources. In his recent book *here is where we meet*, John Berger writes about that period in the last ice age when there were many species of animals which are now extinct, such as mammoths and aurochs. Cro-Magnon lived among the animals, but it was the animals who were the keepers of the world. And, Berger notes, Cro-Magnons lived "with fear and amazement" in a culture that faced many mysteries and lasted for approximately 20,000 years, whereas our culture, of only two or three centuries, "instead of facing mysteries, persistently tries to outflank them."

Maybe Charlotte sees in animals that quality of being prepared to face mysteries. Animals have a kind of presentness that allows them to experience, acknowledge and accept things, without trying to analyze, outwit or bypass them. The other day I asked Charlotte what she thought was the difference between animals and humans. She looked very somber, as she contorted her face in concentrated thought. She's such a pretty child, yet often her large dark eyes seem full of ancient wisdom, which gives her the appearance of an aged dwarf. When she didn't immediately produce an answer, I told her I'd heard a story from a long-time neighbour of Jane Jacobs, that great writer and social critic who died in Toronto recently, about how Jacobs and her brother had, as children, anguished over this question. Finally, they came to the conclusion that animals don't have kitchens and that was the really big difference.

"Yes," Charlotte said, "Animals don't bother with that. They just eat their food. They don't cook it."

We chatted about this for a while, agreeing that animals did have homes, and beds, and neighbourhoods, and so forth, but never kitchens.

"And," I added, "Some people say the difference is that animals are nicer than people."

Charlotte gave me a huge approving smile. "That's what I think too," she nodded.

I'm not as misanthropic as my granddaughter, but it's true that there are too many of us, too many humans. When I think about the future, scenes from the Verdi-induced nightmare return. That swirl of dark-suited courtiers circling around the innocent, luminous Gilda, the darkness radiating inward and obliterating her virtue. The image resonates with me in terms of contemporary human activities, suggesting the kinds of corruption one sees in government offices and public institutions, as well as on the dark streets of our inner cities. I try to turn the image around somehow, and focus not on the word "evil" but on its reverse: "live." That's what the radiation is intended to help me do.

On my last morning in Victoria, there is a final verse from Gerry. He has not missed a day of sending these email ditties. This one, entitled "Wriggleletter," says

So how was Rigoletto?
Did the mad Count get him back?
And did Gilda sing falsetto
When they stuffed her in the sack?
So when you're in your tube today
Just know things could be worse
You could be stuck like Gilda
With Monterone's curse.

He's right. Things could be a lot worse. I'm lucky, in more ways than I can count. I'm well attended by my general practitioner, who seems genuinely to care about me. My surgeon has been humane and communicative in all my contact with him throughout the two surgeries. My oncologist, an intelligent young woman, always treats me as a sensible person who is capable of receiving information and making sound decisions. I've had no side effects from the radiation and they didn't even put me in a tube!

When I leave the Cancer Clinic after my final session, I take stock of all the things that make this a hospitable environment. The cheerful volunteers, the colourful paintings, the overall groundedness of the people and place. The warm slate floors at the entrance, the slightly Japanese look of the high wooden porticos in contrast to the institutional brick, and the lush landscaping that features rock gardens, azaleas and other shrubs. Light streams through the high windows. It feels healthy here.

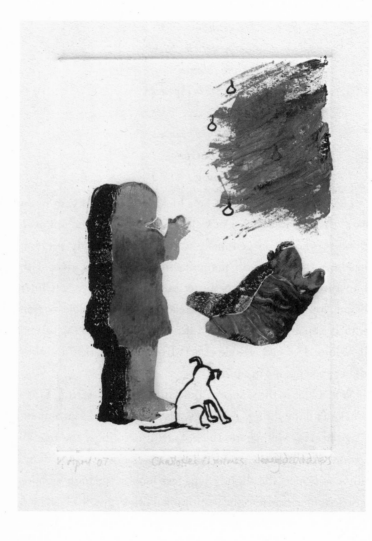

Charlotte's Christmas

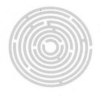

Seasons

I'VE MADE IT through that hard winter, spring and summer, and now the autumn season has officially begun. People keep asking me about my health. I tell them that, as far as I know, I'm well. When I mention that I have a follow-up appointment at the cancer clinic in another few months they ask if I am worried about it. No, I say, I feel fine. The truth is I feel as I did when we had cockroaches years ago in our Montreal apartment. After the exterminator came we couldn't see the cockroaches anymore but at night I would lie awake picturing them crawling around in the cupboards, in the drawers, invisible and increasing.

In the late fall, my husband and I fly to Montreal, and from there set off on train travels to connect with old friends, those people with whom our friendship has endured over decades and despite distance. We also visit people in our family, my niece and her daughter in Ottawa, and my nephew and his family in Toronto. It's wonderful to have these reunions, this labyrinthine journey, winding around in time and space. Such circles of connection and care offer a healing ritual to end this year which began so badly.

In Halifax, I meet up with my friend Jo. She says she's doing well, and she looks more elegant than ever. Recently she endured a round of radiation treatment that she can only describe as like being turned on a spit for 24 hours. Something from Brueghel's *Slaughter of the Innocents*, or at least that was the image she had of the waiting room at the cancer centre. "Head-scarved women with stricken faces bloated from chemo sessions waiting for the axe to fall," she says. Having survived this treatment, Jo is now determined to do everything she wants to do and only what she wants to do. A few days ago she returned from ten days in London. She'll go to Newfoundland for a Tai Chi course next month. After Christmas she's heading off to Jakarta to spend time with her brother.

In Toronto, I visit my old friend and mentor, Connie. Celebrated academic, distinguished editor and author of several critical books, anthologies, textbooks, essays and short stories, Connie is famously indefatigable and full of grace in every challenge she takes on. Having just completed six sessions of chemotherapy for ovarian cancer, she's now preparing to spend some time in Mexico where she'll entertain successive rounds of visitors, while flying back to Toronto as needed to maintain her breakneck schedule of professional commitments.

One of the important reasons for this trip was to see Jo and Connie. I wanted to know just how they were prevailing now that their worlds were transformed by cancer, and I learned that cancer, like bereavement, affects everyone differently. We each have our own ways of responding to the likelihood of a shortened lifespan. My slow journey across the country, wanting to connect with the family and friends who have been so important in my life, seems very pale, contrasted with the energetic ventures of my friends. I know they'll pack a lot more into whatever time is left.

My husband tells me he learned a new "fact" from watching morning television in our hotel room (something he would never do at home, if only because at home we have no cable and the one channel we get is pretty dodgy). He heard a scientist explain that if you could measure time as it exists with one person sitting still, quiet and inactive, compared with another person who is running around wildly, you'd find that the lengths of time were actually different.

What does that mean except that at some moments we experience time as racing along, while at others time drags? When we return home from our travels, it feels as though we've been away for months but, while traveling, our journey seemed to go very quickly. Sometimes time deepens, and sometimes it races, and, in the end, it all turns into timelessness.

And now the Christmas season is upon us again. A year ago, Charlotte and I were both ill at Christmas. It was not the best of times. This year I want to make Christmas as magical as it was when I was a child. I plan to boycott the getting and spending, and focus again on Christmas carols, decorations, a few traditions, a lot of generosity but not a lot of presents.

Charlotte is terribly excited on Christmas Eve, and so she doesn't get to sleep until after eleven, which means that she sleeps in on Christmas Day. I have never, never, in my whole life slept in on Christmas Day, I tell my husband. He and I rise very early to turn on the tree lights, clear away the cookies and milk left for Santa and his reindeer, and make sure that the scene in our living room is well set for Charlotte's Christmas morning. We put Handel's *Messiah* on and settle in to read for a little while, waiting for the others to awaken, but finally, eager to get on with things, we even start ringing jingle bells outside Charlotte's door and still she sleeps on until well after nine, by which time even her late-sleeping parents have arisen.

Finally Charlotte emerges from her room, rubbing her eyes. "I must have overslept," she says, catching sight of the full stockings stacked up by the tree. Sitting down beside our dog, Victor, she slowly opens the presents Santa brought for him before getting to her own. At last we all begin the lengthy process of opening and passing around each gift. It is a gentle day, with afternoon naps all around and a festive but low-key dinner.

After dinner, we sing some carols and lounge in the living room, admiring the Christmas tree. It's a well-shaped tree, just the right size to hold all the historical decorations, a nice showing of coloured lights, and a great scattering of red birds that I bought in memory of the tree my husband and I had for our first Christmas together. On that long-ago tree, the only decorations were a bunch of birds I'd constructed out of coloured paper, and a lot of round cookies with faces made of raisins, nuts and cherries. We didn't have much money, and I'd decided to recreate a childhood story in which a poor family had no Christmas tree but hung a few cookies on a tree outside their window and in the morning found that the tree was magnificently decorated with an array of singing birds.

My childhood Christmas trees were less organic and much gaudier than the one now in our living room. They were dense with decorations, looped with shredded tin-foil garlands, and covered with tinsel icicles. But those decorations were carefully removed and boxed up each year, and there was always the business, after Christmas, of removing the tiny strands of tinsel, icicle by icicle, strand by strand, painstakingly untangling them and carefully packing them up for use again the next year. Although they cost very little, it wouldn't have occurred to my parents that the tinsel decorations could be discarded and replaced with new ones.

Times change, and the years curve around. Another Christmas. Another new year. What lies ahead now appears more hopeful than it did during last year's bleak midwinter. I am apparently cancer-free, and have entered this year ten pounds lighter than when I began it. I'm walking more, drinking less, and trying to be a healthier person. For the first time in our marriage, my husband and I went to bed before midnight on New Year's Eve, and let the new year slip in while we slept. I've only made five resolutions for this new year:

- Drink eight glasses of water each day.
- Walk a mile a day.
- Avoid airplane travel.
- Avoid eating meat.
- Memorize a Shakespeare sonnet every week. This will serve me well if I am to spend a lot of time in medical treatment, and it will also help me figure out how to deal with growing old.

Two for me. Two for the planet. One to help to find a way through everything, whatever everything turns out to be.

We've had astonishing storms in British Columbia this winter, hurricane force at times, with power outages, trees falling on houses, ferries being cancelled, and a generally biblical sense of things coming to an end. These historic storms caused devastation of a sort we have not seen before. Vancouver's Stanley Park lost more than a thousand trees, some that had been there for over two hundred years, from before the park was declared a park. A friend in a secluded Oak Bay neighbourhood lost an enormous and handsome old tree and others on Hornby Island endured weeks without power or water. Strangely, we on tiny

Protection Island, in the middle of all this, were spared. No fallen trees, no power outages, no telephone wires down.

Maybe next time it will be our turn. Things have a way of turning around. *To everything there is a season, and a time to every purpose under the heaven.* Turn, turn, turn, Pete Seeger added, in the lyrics to his song, emphasizing the circularity of all things. And he added one other line to the words of Ecclesiastes: *I swear it's not too late.*

I've noticed that, in these end-of-times times, most of my friends seem to be writing something, as though we're all afraid that perhaps it is too late, and we're desperate to leave a record of how things were on our planet at this particular time. We hope, perhaps, that somewhere, sometime, some creature in another universe might possibly care to know.

Here's a metaphor for human behaviour on our planet. On our island, there's a shortage of dock space for boaters to use. There's one rotten old dock which has been falling apart for years, and everyone who uses it has had a fall at one time or another. Everyone says that one of these days there's going to be a really bad accident. It could be a disaster. The owner has shown no sign of fixing the dock, and nobody else is going to fix it, because it's not their dock. But there's nowhere else to go, and their boats are moored to this dock. So everyone waits for the inevitable disaster that will destroy the dock. The dock to which the boats are moored.

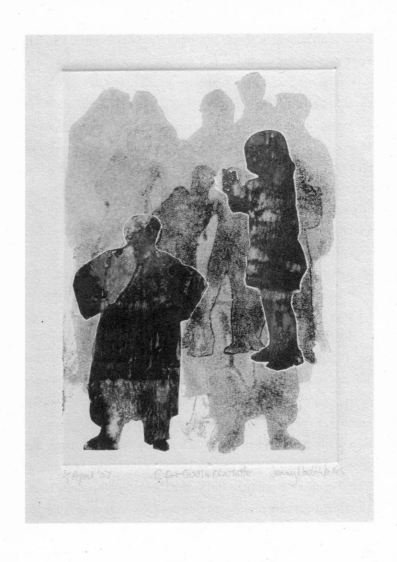

C for Carol and Charlotte

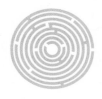

The C-Word

"What's the greatest letter of all?" I ask my granddaughter, Charlotte, as I have done at regular intervals, from the time she began to talk. "The letter C," she replies, without fail. She knows just why this is, offering an ever-expanding list of the letter's attributes. C is for Charlotte, and Carol, and Christmas. And for cookies, candies, cats, carousels and carnivals. "C" is the first letter Charlotte learned to write, and Middle C is the first note she learned on the piano.

These days, for me, the letter C means another word—"the C-Word," which usually suggests cancer, and often appears right after the word "dreaded." Why do we use such euphemistic terms, anyway? *The C-Word. The F-Word?* Usually these are merely coy ways of avoiding obscenities. But what is it about the word "cancer" that stops us from saying it out loud? It's just too scary, so we say "the C-Word" or "the Big C." As Rudyard Kipling observed nearly a hundred years ago, "Human nature seldom walks up to the word 'cancer'."

"C" is also for the word "cure," to which cancer victims cling hopefully, but I wonder if the word "cause" isn't more to the point: consumption and contamination. I can't help thinking that the reason more and more people are suffering from cancer has to do with our excessive consumption, and our continuing contamination of this beautiful, small and preciously green planet. I can't help thinking that my lifelong addictions to excessive food, drink and sloth have contributed to the development of my cancer. The contaminants in the air and water haven't helped. Nor the thoughtless practices of the science-loving 'fifties of my youth. Looking back, it's hard to believe how much time we spent staring, fascinated, at the bones in our feet, courtesy of the x-ray machines in shoe departments. Or the amount of time we spent spraying everything in sight with carcinogens. Here's how things went in those days:

- My father sprayed DDT on the apple and peach trees
- My mother sprayed fabric-protectors on the chesterfield
- We used lemon-scented furniture spray on the table and chairs
- My girlfriends and I sprayed starch on our white cotton blouses
- We sprayed powdered deodorants under our arms

- We kept our beehive hairdos in place with scented hairspray
- We painted rooms with spray paint
- We cleaned windows and ovens with sprays that made you cough
- We killed insects with sprays
- We freshened our mouths with sprays

Very little was left unsprayed during my adolescence. And we tossed all the empty spray cans into the landfill.

The small island on which I live has dirt roads and very few cars. We have wildflowers and a diversity of birds, including eleven Great Blue Heron nests. Our seasons are characterized by the trilling chorus of frogs that announces the arrival of spring and the parade of sea lions that sails by in the late fall. Some mornings, when I look out my window and see the blue heron make his majestic way across the pebbled beach, I think I know what E.O. Wilson means when he says we should ascend to nature (and not away from it, as some fundamentalists may prefer) to a better world. Yet the lives my husband and I live are, for the most part, unnatural. We live outside of nature, and much of what we do is destructive of it.

We make an effort, of course. We recycle as much as we can, through the efforts of a young neighbour who drives her golf-cart around the island picking things up and taking them by boat to the recycling centre. On our island there are dedicated volunteers who rid the public spaces of invasive species that threaten the diversity of the wildlife. I try to do my part by ripping up the English ivy that is spreading across our property, but I can't help feeling that it is I, not the ivy, that is truly invasive.

This weekend we are visiting our family in Vancouver, and I am again off to the labyrinth, in quest of the only meditation I know that helps me to sort out my thoughts. Today it is a silent walk, with no music, and the only others here are two women, one older and one younger. Something about their movement and the circular patterns of our journey reminds me of the figures in Jennifer's prints. Without making any eye contact, one of us steps aside when another needs to pass, or when our paths cross. I'm usually ready to step aside, because this allows a pause, and a chance to look around and look again at some of the photographs and paintings on the wall. But when I step back in I panic for a moment, worrying that I may not be on the right path. Maybe this time I have really lost my way, I think, but then I remind myself just to stay on the path, trust it, and remember that the aim is not to reach the centre of the labyrinth but to reach the centre of oneself.

There is a Portuguese prayer to the *Divino Espirito Santo* that P.K. Page once told me was the only one that meant something to her. It is, simply, *Clarifica me*. That's what I'm after. I am trying to clarify my thoughts about the possibility of the cancer returning or the possibility that it will not, which is really no less frightening. Death lies ahead in either scenario, and that's the thing I need to face. But I feel less fearful of death than I did when I first learned I had cancer. Old age can be as scary as dying. Kurt Vonnegut had it right when he said, "When Hemingway killed himself he put a period at the end of his life; old age is more like a semicolon." There are institutions filled with old people sitting around all day, waiting for the other shoe to fall.

When I reach the centre of the labyrinth, I remain alone in the rosette for some time, waiting for awareness. I think of my friend Connie. She has just learned that her cancer has returned, and she confronts whatever lies ahead with such courage and cheerfulness that she breaks the hearts of all who know and love her.

> *C is for Constance,*
> *Cheerful and clever,*
> *We wish she would live on*
> *For ever and ever.*

If anyone can defy the odds, it is Connie. But none of us can live forever, and who would want it? Swift's Struldbrugs aptly warn us against the desire to prolong life. "Opinionative, peevish, covetous, morose, vain, talkative," these old people are cut off from pleasure, and the least miserable among them are those who have entirely lost their memories.

What's less easy to accept is the aggressive breast cancer that has struck my son-in-law's younger sister, Charlotte's aunt. It doesn't make any sense. Sharon is a healthy, happy, active and attractive young woman in her early forties with no family history of cancer and no lifestyle risk factors. In addition to their busy work activities and their two wonderful children, Sharon and her husband have a small farm and recently acquired two horses and a donkey, along with their two dogs. Their world seemed close to idyllic when, from a somewhat routine check-up with her general practitioner, Sharon suddenly found herself faced with the news that she'd have to undergo a double mastectomy; she is now just concluding what's been a very difficult six-month course of chemotherapy. Sharon has responded to the temporary shattering of everyday life with humour, intelligence and admirable resilience, regularly logging her progress on a blog, making jokes about how devastatingly cute her wig is and how incredibly well-endowed she expects to be post-reconstruction. Her husband and her children have been magnificent throughout it all, constant, caring and supportive, and her family and friends have rallied around, creating one of those windows through which one is able to see the best of human behaviour. Such windows offer us all a glimpse of who and what really matters in our lives.

But it's all a little easier to accept when one is older. At a certain age, we move our thoughts away from our own lives and begin to think of life itself. Many people have written about how illness can provide the opportunity for personal growth, and how an experience with cancer has allowed them to face their own mortality, get in touch with their deepest feelings, and set new and better boundaries in their personal relationships. It can be "a wake-up call," as they say. Facing death can also highlight the preciousness of the time remaining so that one may, like Scrooge on Christmas Day, find it possible to seize the moment to repair wrongs and do good.

I walk back to the hotel, stopping for a moment by English Bay, my mind full of questions about human nature and our inability to live in harmony with the natural world. We have made a mess of things, caused harm to other species and to the planet that we have not been able to repair. Too late we are beginning to learn that there is no such thing as "junk," no such place as "away." It is all here, and always with us. Yet, even in the midst of this huge city, one can see small microwildernesses. Little tufts of grass creep out between the rocks along the beach. At the edge of the water, there are bits of shell and seaweed that the ocean washes in. Despite the damage we do, the earth has huge powers of resilience.

Last year in Montreal, I saw an exhibition by French landscape architect Gilles Clément in which he presented his concept of the *tiers paysage*, the Third Landscape, which derives from the pre-revolutionary French designation of the Third Estate. The Third Landscape, Clément says, is a space that expresses neither power, nor submission to power. His exhibition celebrates those urban spaces in which ecological diversity continues through a combination of natural processes and limited human intervention. As in the images of the Green Man who has leaves and vines springing from his mouth, these small surges of natural vitality in the midst of a busy city reassure us that life carries on.

In my mind are echoes of the concert we heard last night, the celebratory sound of Vivaldi's *Gloria in D Major*. D major, once called "the key of glory," because of its bright sound. It's the natural key of the trumpet, and also allows the maximum number of open strings on the violin. The spirit of the Vivaldi Chamber Choir singing *Gloria*, that joyful hymn of praise and worship, is fitting for the delight I feel seeing small green sprigs shooting up from cracks in the pavement's concrete.

Just outside the hotel I see an art car bedecked with every imaginable kind of junk: a whole line of old faucets, several dozen jeweled angels, scores of hearts and flowers, miniature cars and bells and whistles of every possible sort. From a window on the right side of the car, an enormous stuffed tiger is emerging and a blue and white plush rabbit peers out from the back window. On the hood of a car is a small golden pool, boasting a real, splashing waterfall in which several angels bathe and from which an orca whale is leaping. The car is covered with messages. BEYOND BOUNDARIES is appliquéd in big blue letters. *Peace is a gift we can give to one another*, says one message. *Be wise*, says another. *Let go, let flow. Let there be light.*

Yes, indeed. I laugh out loud at the splendid incongruity of this creation. The Buddhas and the bunnies, and the angels bathing with the whales! In the midst of all the chaos and confusion, and corruption and contamination, and the plague and the pestilence, and the garbage and the glory, and the junk and the joy, let there be light. *Fiat lux!*